Throw Like A Girl:

How Good Coaches Transform Girls Into Successful Women

How Sports Empower Girls to Excel In Life

By Rebecca L. Williams
(Coach R LaShun Williams)

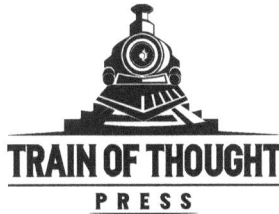

TRAIN OF THOUGHT
PRESS

ISBN: 978-0-9861485-4-5
Library of Congress Number: 2016944471

Summary: Women's Basketball Coach R LaShun Williams gives advice on how to use sports to empower girls to excel in life

Connie Johnston
Train of Thought Press
2275 Huntington Drive, Suite 306
San Marino, CA 91108
TrainofThoughtPress.com

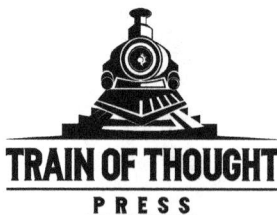

TRAIN OF THOUGHT
P R E S S

Table of Contents

Introduction

I always knew coaching was important, but I didn't realize exactly how important until a girl named Kelley came into my life.

I had coached girls who needed my encouragement before her. After all, junior high is tough. Kids rush into the middle school years with bright eyes but few exit the other side of the gauntlet without scars. I've seen plenty of stooped shoulders. Downcast eyes. Girls crippled by self-doubt.

But Kelley was different. She had good self-esteem and confidence, and knew what it meant to be a team player. She didn't look like a girl who needed any extra support. However, one day while she went out for a bike ride with her brother as her father was jogging, a drive-by shooter gunned down her father. She watched her father bleed to death on the sidewalk.

Her father was Northwestern University Coach Ricky Byrdsong. His killer was white supremacist Benjamin Smith; Kelley's father was one of twelve victims of Smith's hate crime shooting spree.

As you can imagine, everyone around Kelley was focused on the grotesque details of that horrific hate crime — *so* focused that Kelley's needs as a ten-year-old girl were overlooked. Not because people didn't love her, but because they were so outraged at the nature of the crime that the desire to do something about a bigger problem overshadowed the very real needs of a ten-year-old girl trying to process the death of her precious father.

Kelley needed me to rise up and coach in a way I'd never done before.

That's when I realized the role a coach could play in a young girl's life.

That's when I recognized my true purpose.

It's also the year I truly recognized that coaching is about more than winning. In the two decades I've been coaching I've brought teams to the championships 10 times and won the championships 8 times. Trust me: I like to win as much as anyone. I'm competitive. I demand excellence from my players. I'm a tough coach.

But Kelley Byrdsong and the girls who followed taught me that coaching is about so much more than just winning or losing a tournament.

The techniques you learn in this book will help you win games. However, through my two decades of coaching and training in youth basketball, I have learned that life coaching is essential for success both on and off the court. I'm not just going to teach you how to coach a winning team. I want to show you how to impact young women for a lifetime.

Why You Matter

I don't know how you ended up coaching or what motivated you to read this book, but I'm glad you've taken it on. Thank you!

Maybe you signed up because you want to spend more time with your own child or you want to be a role model to the kids in your community.

Maybe you're a teacher, and every teacher in your school has to contribute, so coaching this team is your way of fulfilling that obligation.

Maybe you were stuck with this position because nobody else would do it.

Or perhaps you are one of the rare individuals who realize that coaching sports is one of the most effective ways to inspire and change young women. (I love it when that's the case!)

Whatever the reason, you are now in a position of power and influence. Most importantly, you have the opportunity to change lives. Congratulations! You've taken the first step. I'm excited to teach you how to make the most of this valuable opportunity.

A Little About Me

My name is Rebecca LaShun Williams (although my players call me "Coach LaShun" or "Ma"). I've witnessed firsthand how much good and bad coaches affect the young women they lead.

I have a bachelor's degree from Gustavus Adolphus College in pre-law and psychology and over 20 years of experience as a professional business consultant within the human resources field. As such, I have a strong understanding of human behavior.

I am also a certified professional coach with over 20 years of experience and act as an ambassador for the International Coaching Academy (ICA).

More importantly, I've spent over 20 years with my players, coaching basketball. I know what it takes to be a great coach. And most importantly, I understand why our young women need good coaches — coaches who want to make a difference.

More Than Just a Coach

To tell the truth, I was sick of coaching at the time Kelley came into my life. I was thinking about throwing in the towel. I was tired of the politics, pressure and frustration with parents who either didn't show up or tried to coach from the sidelines.

Then Kelley was placed on my team and I saw how much I truly had to offer. This girl was in need. Not just for a basketball coach, but for a strong adult presence and support.

Today Kelley calls me her second mom. She is now a college graduate, working as a life coach for adolescents. Her light shines brightly. I'm proud to be a part of her success story.

But Kelley is not the only one. Millions of girls are also in need of inspiring coaches who can teach them how to win both on and off the court.

Take these principles to heart and you'll celebrate more than a championship win. You'll celebrate the victories of confident young women and the other women they influence, all because they had a coach who cared enough to do the job right.

You can and should be that coach.

Ready to get started? Let's go!

Chapter One: Hear the Cry of America's Young Women

It's a great day to be a girl in America... or is it? While this is a time of opportunity, we have a long way to go in building a strong workforce of confident, empowered young women.

Guess who is positioned to influence these young women? You already know the answer. It's you, the coach.

The Jungle of Adolescence

If you've forgotten what it feels like to be an adolescent girl, I urge you to take a walk down the halls of a junior high school during passing period. Listen to the babble of voices. Watch the body language of the kids. Take a good whiff of the malodorous scent of hormones percolating in those growing bodies.

Adolescence is rough.

A survey of 3,000 children conducted by the American Association of University Women concluded that although 60 percent of girls reported feeling confident at age nine (when first surveyed), self-esteem plummeted during the middle school and high school years. By the time those same girls reached high school, only 29 percent reported still feeling confident.

Take a look at these statistics and you'll quickly see that this is only the tip of the iceberg:

- According to DoSomething.org, seven in ten girls believe that they are not good enough or don't measure up (when thinking about their appearance, academic performance, friendships or relationships with family members).
- According to the Dove Campaign, 92 percent of girls would like to change how they look (weight issues are the top concerns listed).
- According to *The Triple Bind* by Steven Hinshaw, one in four girls is clinically diagnosed with one or more of the following conditions: depression, an eating disorder, self harming or another mental and/or emotional disorder. These numbers only include those who are actually diagnosed. Many more go undiagnosed and untreated.
- According to the National Institute on Media and the Family, 53 percent of thirteen-year-old girls are unhappy with their bodies. That number jumps to 78 percent by the time girls reach age seventeen.

There's no doubt about it. Our young women are struggling emotionally.

How does that struggle affect them as they grow into adulthood?

Women in the Real World

We're pretty good at parroting the line that America is the land of gender equality, but women still struggle to get the same pay and opportunities as men. Check out some more statistics to get a clear picture of the world into which we're sending our young women:

- According to the Center for American Women and Politics, only three women have served as state governors in the history of our country. In contrast, our population has elected 2,319 male governors.
- According to *CNN Money*, only three percent of Fortune 500 CEOs are women.
- According to the Inter-Parliamentary Union, 89 countries have more women in national legislative positions than we do.
- According to *Advertising Age*, only three percent of all creative directors (employed by advertising agencies) are women, and women hold only three percent of high-powered positions in the mainstream media.
- According to *The Economist*, while 29 percent of American businesses are owned by women, businesses owned by women only account for four percent of total American business revenues.

Looks like we've got a long way to go, America. Fortunately, coaches have a unique opportunity to make a dent in this problem. Yes, you as a coach can make a significant impact on the young women on your team. Don't believe me? Read on.

How Do Sports Fit Into the Big Picture?

While family environment and other influences are indeed important, participation in youth sports greatly increases a girl's chances of succeeding in a wide variety of ways both in adolescence and in her adult life. Once again, let the numbers do the talking:

Each year approximately 36,000,000 kids between the ages of five and eighteen play organized sports. Broken down into genders, 66 percent of boys and 52 percent of girls play organized sports. The benefits of participation in sports is compelling.

For example, female high school athletes (when compared to non-athletes) are:

- 92 percent less likely to get involved with drugs.
- 80 percent less likely to get pregnant.
- Three times more likely to graduate.

There are many established benefits of participation in youth sports, including the following:

- Participation in sports builds and maintains healthy bones, muscles and joints.
- Controls weight, reduces fat and improves overall health.
- Positively affects aspects of personal development such as self-esteem, goal-setting and capacity for leadership.
- Assists with development and improvement of cognitive skills, including:
  - Improved academic achievement, including grades and standardized test scores.
  - Enhanced attitude and behavior, including better concentration, attention and classroom behavior.

But does participation in youth sports really translate into better success as adults?

Studies conclude that:

- Youths that play sports are eight times as likely to be active at age twenty-four as adolescents who do not play sports.

- Women who played high school sports were 73 percent more likely to graduate from college within six years of completing high school than those who did not play sports. (This percentage holds up even when we account for socioeconomic challenges.)

- Approximately 73 percent of corporate executives played sports as children or adolescents.

- Youths that participated in organized sports are more likely to engage in adult involvement in community activities for their entire lifetime.

- Teenagers who played sports developed stronger leadership skills, worked better in teams and demonstrated more confidence than teens who did not participate in athletics. As adults, they demonstrated "significantly higher levels of leadership, self-confidence and self-respect" than their non-athletic peers.

Where You Come In

While participation in sports is beneficial, the quality of coaching is a key factor in maximizing positive effects.

You've probably noticed that the world has come to recognize sports in the realm of everyday life. In the corporate world, job listings often mention "team player" as a requirement. Your co-workers may be referred to as your team members and managers are often referred to as your coach. A lot of people refer to their spouse and children as their team.

Surely you've seen the parallels.

At work:
- Coach — Your manager
- Teammates — Your co-workers
- Referees — Your executive staff

This application of sports analogies is common because many of the principles and skills learned in sports can be applied to success in life overall.

When you coach a team, you step into important shoes. In the following chapters, you will learn how to use each aspect of coaching to teach your players how to develop habits that will translate into winning both on and off the court.

Chapter Two: What Makes a Good Coach Good

Before I get into details about how to translate sports skills into life skills, I want to talk to you about you. Why? Because your attitude matters more than any techniques or drills I can possibly teach you.

What you do and say makes a difference. In fact, 81.5 percent of the participation in sports amongst six to twelve-year-old youths is directly correlated to the behavior of the coach.

What does that mean? If you are a good coach, you will have a successful team and you will have players return the following year. Why? Because you inspired them. You made them believe they could do it. You helped them grow.

If you're a lazy, neglectful or downright abusive coach, you may or may not win the season. However, win or lose, you will lose players because you discouraged the kids.

Why Your Behavior Matters

The kids on your team may come from broken homes (the Family Research Council reports that 55 percent of teens live in broken homes and 30 percent of kids live in single-parent households). They may not have support from their parents, and not necessarily because their parents don't want to be there (although that happens, too), but because their parents are either working or busy with other family demands. The kids on your team may not have basic needs met or may have self-esteem problems.

As their coach, you may become the person who writes recommendation letters, protects a child from peer pressure, supplies the child with the resources they need or even helps them fill out college applications. If you take coaching seriously, you may become a second mom/dad or even a replacement guardian.

At the very least, you become a role model. You become the person who embodies what it is to be a leader. A respectable adult, deserving of admiration. You can help those young women determine who they want to be when they grow up.

But what makes a good coach good and a bad coach bad? Read on to find out.

You Know You're a Good Coach If... You Prioritize Healthy Self-Esteem

In my 19 years of coaching, I've seen this again and again: the biggest problem these girls face is low self-esteem.

Take Sariah, for example. (The girl's actual name has been changed to protect the player.)

Sariah joined my team as a fifth grader. She was overweight, had health problems and had never played basketball. When the ball was passed to her, she shied away from it; when the basket was open, she hesitated until the window of opportunity had passed. She ran from the ball instead of to it and she looked for opportunities to hang back instead of getting in on the action.

It quickly became evident to me that Sariah's problem was a lack of confidence. She saw herself as fat. Incapable. Uncoordinated. Unworthy of even being on the court. She believed she would fail, and as a result, she struggled — both on and off the court.

Sariah was definitely not the only one. While each season there are usually a few bright shining stars who walk onto the court already confident and self-assured, most of the girls I've coached don't realize their potential — at least not at the beginning of the season. By the end of the season, I've built up their self-esteem to the point where they believe in themselves.

Once a girl believes in herself, you can challenge her to improve specific skills. In fact, the very challenges you offer her (and the growth she experiences when she accepts the challenges) build upon that foundational level of self-confidence. However, if you challenge a girl to change without first showing that you believe in her, you may crush her. It's a delicate balance — a fine line to walk.

Thanks to Sariah, I've come up with an exercise I now do at the beginning of every season.

Have each girl stand up and introduce herself. Then pass out paper and pencils and ask the girls to write down the answers to the following questions:

- Where do you currently see yourself as a basketball player?
- How do you believe you can contribute to the team?
- How do you want to develop as a player?

We discuss these answers at the following practice. The girls who are comfortable speaking in front of the group read their answers aloud; the others hand their papers in to me and I help them share.

Then we discuss the core issues these questions address, making it clear that I want to get to know each girl individually. I spend time with their answers, responding positively and with specific encouragement. I don't let them get away with vague answers but instead help them see that even as new players, they can contribute. In fact, I communicate (with respect and dignity) that I expect them to contribute and that I believe they will find their place on the team.

After every girl has discussed her hopes for growth and contribution, I talk about how important it is for us to work as a team. I discuss the importance of working together to help every team member grow. Not everyone will be the top scoring player on the team — that's not possible! But they can be the top rebounder or the best defensive player or the player with the most hustle. They could even play the role of motivating other players to work harder when they are down on themselves. As a coach, it is important to make sure everyone knows her role on the team. However, you must also make sure they understand that regardless of the particular role they play, every girl plays a vital part in helping the team succeed.

I talk about how important it is to find your strengths and to use them for the good of the entire team, and how we can't afford to have anyone hanging back. We all need to find what we can do and then do it to the best of our ability.

After this discussion, during which I express my excitement about each and every player, I have the girls write 10 positive things about themselves.

You may be thinking: what about drills? What about physical fitness? You're wasting time talking with the girls and having them write out lists of things they like about themselves?

This is what you need to recognize: most kids cannot think of 10 things they like about themselves. That's how low their self-esteem is.

And that's why it's crucial to invest time fostering healthy self-esteem at the beginning of the season. *Before* they make embarrassing mistakes on the court. (Because it will happen.) Before they miss a key shot. (That will happen, too.) Before they dribble the ball on their foot, sending it rolling out of bounds. (You know that will happen as well.)

You have to get ahead of the self-esteem problem right away.

So make them write down 10 things they like about themselves. Don't let them get away with only 6. Then talk about how important it is to believe in themselves. I always say, "If you don't believe in yourself, I promise you, no one in this world will." I describe the potential I see in each of them and how I look forward to working with them to help them be the best player they can be.

By the way, Sariah was on my team for four years. She lost weight, fell in love with basketball and became a key player. She is now a starting player for her high school team. She also writes and recites poetry on stage and is preparing to go to college.

You Know You're a Good Coach If... You Teach Them Not to Fear Failure

I always tell my kids, "If you miss a million shots, shoot a million and one."

Kids are afraid to try and fail, but if they never try, they'll never succeed. You cannot succeed without trying and risking failure.

I tell them, "You only fail if you don't try. You don't fail if you try and miss. Just shoot again. And if you miss, shoot again, and again, and again. Eventually, you will get it, and once you do, you'll figure out what it takes to get the basket over and over again. Soon it will feel natural to get the basket and the fear of failure will disappear."

"But to get to that point, you have to shoot and miss a lot. If you're not willing to shoot and miss, you'll never get to the point where you get the shot on a regular basis."

When discussing this with the girls, I often quote Wayne Gretzky: "You miss 100 percent of the shots you don't take." This makes the point and gets them to laugh at the same time because of course you can't make a shot you didn't let fly.

It's easier to say this than to actually get the girls to do it. Why? Because they are so afraid of failing in front of other people. The feeling of failure is so dangerous to them that they'd rather not try at all, or only try the minimum number of times.

How do you overcome this? You have to remove the stigma of missing a shot.

Talk about how everybody misses shots, and talk about how important practice is. Let them know that practicing — and missing shots — is the only way to get better. Then, when you've got them doing drills and they're doing lay ups and that girl misses and looks like she didn't even really try, talk about how trying is what matters. Have the girls shoot over and over and over and over. Make it okay to miss a shot — as long as they shoot again.

I always say, "If you're open and in your range, let it go. You have four teammates on the court with you. If you miss, it is their job to get the rebound and put it in. The team will help you; you need to trust in yourself and your teammates. How will you ever score if you never shoot?"

Once they overcome their fear of failure, they'll try, and trying is essential for succeeding.

You Know You're a Good Coach If... Every Team Member Feels Valued

I know you've got your star athletes. Every team has them. It's tempting to put your focus on those kids and ignore the ones who seem unmotivated, unskilled or discouraged.

I challenge you to resist that temptation and to deliberately celebrate every team member.

Give all the kids the same assignments, not just the star players. Play up the potential of every player. Then watch them to see where they fit in on the team and start guiding them to succeed in their particular role. Emphasize that every position is important and has value, and then work to make sure the player feels valuable for performing in that position.

You will also notice that some kids have a chip on their shoulder or think they are the superstars. Some will make it obvious that they think the other players aren't as valuable as they are.

You need to counteract this kind of attitude. Do not tolerate teasing, taunting, bullying or disrespect towards any player.

I've found that team-building activities are essential for building unity and help diffuse this attitude. Schedule teamwork exercises and activities such as the following:

- Ice cream or pizza party
- A picnic at the beach, pool or park
- Human knot
- Pass the hula hoop
- Relay races
- Watermelon-eating race
- Wheelbarrow race
- Team outing (to watch another team play or to do something fun)
- Pass the egg (with a spoon)

If you aren't familiar with the activities listed here or need to look up more, try Googling "team-building activities for kids".

The more you can develop a sense of "we are all important" and "we are in this together," the more success you will experience.

Your goal? To develop a team attitude where kids even give up a chance to shoot and give it to the weakest player so she has a chance to score. By building a team that views every player as valuable, you build a strong, unified force. A force to be reckoned with!

You Know You're a Good Coach If... You Meet the Needs of the Kids

If a child doesn't know where her next meal is coming from, she can't concentrate. If all the other kids have new shoes but one kid doesn't have shoes or gear, she will be too embarrassed to play well. If a kid has lost a family member, she won't be able to focus.

It's your job to notice these things. Over the years, I have:

- Given kids rides to and from practices and games.
- Provided (or organized) snacks for the team just to make sure everyone got fed.
- Taken kids out for a meal after practices and games because I knew they weren't eating properly at home.
- Given players clothing, shoes and gear.
- Given out my cell number and texted the kids to inspire them and make sure they know someone cares.
- Helped them with homework and job and college applications.
- Flown from Chicago to places like D.C. to support former players when they are struggling. One of my

former players' father even calls me his baby's momma.

Here's another story for you. One year, I found out that one of the girls on my junior high school team lived in a bad part of town. She even had a bullet hole in her apartment front door from a shooting that happened while she was standing in front of her home.

Although she was an amazing kid with extremely good grades and impressive basketball skills, she didn't have proper eating habits or gear. I watched her give her all, on the court and off. After seeing how much effort she put into being an excellent player and student, I talked to the overseeing staff and got support to give this girl what every basketball player wants — a pair of Jordans. We also gave her dry fit shirts and socks. We did this privately, of course, so as to not embarrass her and to ensure nobody got jealous.

It's up to you to see the needs of your players and to get those needs met. Does she need a friend? Buddy her up with another player you know will take her under their wing. Does she need clothes? Buy her some or find someone who will donate good clothes to her. Take her to Goodwill for a shopping trip, if nothing else. Is she struggling in school? Stay with her after school and help her finish her homework.

When you show your players that you see their needs and are willing to meet them, they will be loyal. They will work hard for a coach of that caliber.

You Know You're a Good Coach If... Your Players Know You Care

Kids need to know someone cares. That means you've got to show up to practice, the games and beyond.

You've seen coaches who are there in body but not in spirit. You know what I mean. They haven't thought through a plan for practice. They bark at the players and check their cell phones instead of truly caring about the game.

Refuse to be that coach. Instead, be the coach who comes prepared and excited for every practice and every game. Get to know your kids and make sure they know you care about the team. Invest yourself emotionally. The kids will feel it, and they also will invest in the team.

Once you do this, you'll find yourself emotionally attached to your players. I even go to the kids' games after they've graduated from my league. There's nothing like watching a proud high school player whom you coached when she was in junior high. When she makes a good play, she'll look into the stand just to see if you noticed. The sense of pride you'll both share is worth the extra effort.

You Know You're a Good Coach If... You Teach the Kids to Find Solutions

I tell my kids, "There will be obstacles, but there are ways around any obstacle."

Then we talk strategy. What to do if someone blocks you. What to do if you're outside shooting range and nobody is free. What to do when your teammate misses a shot.

I expose them to the delight of finding hidden opportunities. This turns obstacles into adventures and teaches them perseverance. By teaching them how to find solutions, I'm teaching them how to fish (instead of just feeding them for a day).

You Know You're a Good Coach If... You Care as Much as the Kids Do

Are you as excited about the game as the kids are? Or are you slouching on the sidelines, biding your time?

Have someone video you as you coach a game, and then watch the video to see what you look like. You might be surprised by what you see.

I dance on the sidelines when one of my kids scores or makes a good play. I cheer them on, loudly. I clap and hoot and holler.

My kids know that I'm excited about every minute of the game, even if we aren't winning. I'm just as loud and enthusiastic when encouraging a player after she misses a shot or makes a bad play as I am when she succeeds.

Why do I do this? Because I know how important it is to convey my support and positive, constructive guidance when a kid makes a mistake. In fact, this is even more important than celebrating a victory.

When a player makes a mistake on the court, they feel horrible about it. You've been there. Imagine for a moment that you just missed a shot in front of all your peers and parents. You feel awful, right? That is the moment of vulnerability — and also the moment your praise and encouragement means the most. If you help a player believe she can recover from failure and do something to make up for the mistake, you have truly won. This is where the real victories are scored.

Show the kids that you believe in them by doing things such as the following:

- Encourage them to shoot again if they miss a shot.
- Keep them in the game after they make a big mistake (and tell them it's okay).
- Cheer them on when you see them making an effort (regardless of whether or not the effort resulted in tangible results).
- Clap them on the shoulder when you have to take them out of the game (and tell them "good job" or "nice effort" or "you're going to get your game back, don't worry," as is appropriate).
- Assure them that they will figure it out whenever they hit something difficult.

Be passionate beyond what others expect. Your passion is infectious. The kids will feed off your enthusiasm, even when the game isn't going well. Your ability to keep believing in them will help them believe in themselves.

You Know You're a Good Coach If... You Set a Good Example

Kids watch your every move. They see how you respond when someone misses a shot. They search your face for looks of disgust or signs that you have given up on the game. They look from the scoreboard to your face to see if they should keep trying or if it's time to give up.

They will pay especially keen attention to how you interact with each player. Do you favor someone? Does that annoying player get under your skin? How do you react? With maturity or immaturity?

They learn how to interact with the competition by your example, too. Are you intimidated by a team with a good record, or are you confident your team can beat them? Do you hold your head high when the other coach is yelling at the referee? Do you handle yourself with dignity? How do you respond to unruly parents on the sidelines?

They watch during the practice and games, but they'll also watch when they interact with you outside the sports world. How do you greet your partner? Their parents? Your friends? Are you proud of them off the court, or was it just an act when you were in "coach" mode?

My kids call me Momma Hen, Mom, etc. They respect me because I strive to act in an honorable manner at all times. Do the same and you'll win the respect and loyalty of your players.

You Know You're a Good Coach If... You Refuse to Shame Players

I've seen coaches shame a kid for not having gear instead of digging in and finding out what is happening. Do they not have the money for gear? Maybe they need help with organization and being responsible?

Other coaches shame kids on the court as a way to try to motivate them. If you do that, you may crush a girl's self-esteem completely, affecting much more than your season record.

Treat your players with respect, especially when they fail or disappoint. By helping them preserve their dignity, you preserve the dignity of the entire team.

You Know You're a Good Coach If... You Ask Your Players to Do Their Best

I say the same thing before every game: "I don't care if we win or lose; just get out there and give 110 percent. If you have done your best, there is nothing else anyone can ask of you."

Why do I say this?

Because I became a great coach when I stopped trying to win.

My first year coaching, we won four out of seven games.

The next year, we only won one out of seven games, but we won the championship.

Interestingly enough, when I stopped trying to win and focused on making sure every team member grew, we started winning. And once we started winning, we were unstoppable.

I had a bad car accident that almost killed me. It took seven months for me to even walk, but I knew those kids needed me. There were many days when I felt like quitting, especially when I underwent therapy. However, I wanted to show them that recovery is possible. I put my efforts into daily doing my best so that I was ready to coach by the time the season started.

After I did this, I switched my coaching to focus on helping every player do her best. Now I am back to walking, running, dancing, jumping and playing sports. My recovery inspired the kids to believe that it is possible to come back from a significant setback.

In the nine years following my car accident, we won six out of nine championships. One of the years that my team lost the championship, we lost to a team comprised mostly of kids I had previously coached. (Those kids had been ineffective the year prior, but the five starters improved through my time with them at the AAU program.)

This is when I knew for sure I had stumbled upon a coaching secret. If I can help every player perform to her best ability, we are no longer controlled by the scoreboard. Even if we are down, we can play our hearts out in that last quarter and rally to a win. We can do it because we don't stop trying, regardless of what the scoreboard says.

You Know You're a Good Coach If… You Inspire Others to Support the Team

I don't make a lot of money, but what I do have, I devote to the kids. I'm not shy about this. Why? Am I showing off? Nope. I'm inspiring others to also be generous and that benefits everyone.

When people see you taking care of kids and they witness your sincerity, they will start offering to help as well. Bags of clothes, gear, covering costs of other players — when you start meeting the players' needs, other parents and staff members will follow suit. Not only will they contribute material items, but they will start giving in the non-material ways they've witnessed you contributing to the team — time, rides, study groups, friendship, etc. When you give generously, the people around you will also be inspired to give.

You Know You're a Good Coach If... You Adapt to Your Team's Unique Needs

Not all teams are the same. One year I had a team that lost almost every game. They were, quite frankly, a group of inexperienced players who needed time and practice to get better. Now, when I worked with that group of girls the next year, the repeat players were far more prepared for the game, resulting in a terrific year.

I had to adapt my coaching techniques to meet the needs of that inexperienced team so that they would stay positive despite losing a lot of games. That's a tricky line to walk, but I learned how to balance encouragement and challenges, focusing on doing their best (instead of letting the scoreboard dictate how we felt about ourselves). The next year I was able to challenge them more on technique and skills; they were ready for it.

You also will need to adapt to meet the needs of your team and the needs of specific players. Everyone learns differently, is motivated differently and takes feedback differently. It's your job to pay attention to what works and what doesn't work for each player and to be proactive in your approach.

Here's an example: let's say you have two players, one an attention-seeker and one who is very self-conscious. The attention-seeker might be thrilled when you dance on the sidelines as she makes a basket, whereas the self-conscious player might respond better if you congratulate her personally and a little more quietly as she leaves the court.

Likewise, a confident player may be okay with you using her as an example to demonstrate how to do things (in front of the whole team). A shy player might prefer that you talk about something she performed excellently but not respond well if you ask her to get up in front of everyone and model the skill. Pay attention to how your players respond and adjust appropriately. Your flexibility and attention to detail will pay off.

Coaching Basics

I realize many of you may have stumbled into coaching. If so, you might feel like this is a lot to tackle in one season.

Don't get overwhelmed by this list. Instead, get inspired. Find your unique style of coaching and adopt these points into your practices.

The longer you coach, the more you'll learn how to make a difference. As you grow as a coach, your players will also grow. Before you know it, you'll be celebrating victories on and off the court.

As a coach, you get to influence players in many ways. The next three chapters explore how the skills you foster in youth players can translate into lifelong skills.

Chapter Three: How Training Pays Back Dividends

Training.

When you hear that word, what is your first response?

Do you envision players groaning as they start running laps? Maybe you remember doing drills as a kid and you think of training as the worst part of participation in organized sports.

It's true: training is the least glamorous part of the process. However, it is training that truly develops character, more so than participation in the actual games.

Training is where the sweat pours, skills are honed and confidence is built. Training is where personal victories happen.

It's also where girls grow in ways that will positively affect them in work and at home when they become adults.

As a coach, you will want to use training to develop several personal skills in your players.

Teach Them to Be Coachable

One of the most amazing aspects of training for a sport is the way it develops humility. Your players want to win, right? And in order to win, they have to improve their skills, correct? This sets up the perfect situation for you to teach players to accept correction with humility and grace.

Many girls do not have this down yet. They either take correction as criticism (and are crippled by it) or they take offense to it and refuse to learn. Your job is to help your players understand that correction is a part of growth. It is to be expected; it is the only way to improve.

Talk to your players about this concept. Let them know that you will correct them, but that this is an essential part of becoming better as a player. Tell them that they should expect to be corrected, and that there is nothing wrong with being wrong — as long as they are open to learning how to improve.

When you talk to the team before practice begins, tell them that they should be grateful that someone cares enough to push them to improve beyond where they would get on their own. Explain the concept of constructive criticism. It feels like criticism, but it is offered for their own good.

Praise players who are vulnerable enough to recognize they are not perfect. Let them know that you know honest feedback hurts, but that the best response is to accept the correction and to actively work to change bad habits.

Humility is essential for the real world, both at home and at work. How many times have you had to listen to constructive criticism in a work review? What happens if you respond defensively to your spouse? Have you seen a co-worker become absolutely devastated or cause tremendous stress at work because another co-worker pointed out something that needed to be changed?

How can you best teach the girls to become coachable? Talk to them about the importance of understanding learning styles and welcoming the process of learning. Discussing this helps them think about their experience from the perspective of learning and growing. This will diffuse defensiveness and promote openness to instruction.

Let them know that you are also learning from them. Coaching works both ways; coaches learn a lot from their players (and of course players learn from their coaches). If you tell them you are in this together, they will be more open to your guidance.

When teaching them, cushion criticism with assurance that you believe they can grow. Your confidence in them will help them believe in themselves.

The goal is to teach these young women to accept criticism without defensiveness or giving up. Instead, they need to learn how to interpret correction as positive instruction.

Help Them Understand the Application of Philosophies
Each coach has their own fundamental philosophies regarding how they'd like to see their players work together and tackle the training process. Figure out what your basic ground rules are, make those expectations clear and then enforce them so that your players learn how to absorb and respect a philosophy.

Your company does this when you begin to work for them. Each company has its own mission statement, company culture and basic set of expectations regarding professionalism. It's essential that these girls learn how to adapt to a set of philosophical expectations so they know how to do the same when they start working in the real world.

This is also essential for a successful relationship — and for parenting, as well. When you get married and start a family, you will also expect your children to follow your philosophies.

Teaching a philosophy requires talking about it, enforcing rules, disciplining those who do not live up to expectations and embodying the philosophy through your own actions. For example, if your philosophy is that all team players are equals, you cannot show favoritism to the star player. If your philosophy is that players must be respectful and play by the rules, you can't tolerate disrespect between players.

Make sure you identify your philosophical tenets, clearly communicate them to your players and enforce them throughout the season.

Teach Them to Respond to External Motivation
A good coach should be a great motivator — so good that you can make your players believe in your game plan and basic philosophies. You will need to help them believe that they can do anything if they work hard enough at it.

This requires relentless enthusiasm and positivity. You may need to take action to help yourself stay positive and energetic. For example, make sure you eat a good meal, drink plenty of water and get adequate sleep before each practice and game. You need to take care of yourself so you can pour your positive energy into the kids. You will sometimes need to push past circumstances that are out of your control (such as a rough day at work), but by doing so, you will inspire your kids to also push past when they have a rough day at school.

Inevitably, you will sometimes have girls on the team who think it's not cool to be enthusiastic. You may encounter rolling of eyes or sighs. Some kids may try to get out of the harder parts of practice, skimping on laps or crunches or whatever drills you've arranged.

Your challenge is to help them drop the "I'm too cool to do this" attitude and get on board with the team. I've often been complimented by parents who make comments like, "If Coach sees you need that extra push or time, she's the one to give it to you." (Thank you, Tamara! Yes, I do exactly this!)

As you help the girls realize that working hard and showing enthusiasm is good, you will help them build the character necessary for success on the job. They will excel in the workplace if they learn that enthusiasm is valued.

This will also set them up to be positive parents who inspire their children through positivity and hard work instead of through negativity and unnecessary discipline.

Challenge Them to Find Inspiration Within
As the coach, you should be able to inspire your kids to be the greatest students, players and teammates possible. However, you will do them an even greater service if you teach them to learn to find inspiration and internal drive from within.

You know that, as adults, we don't always have a coach cheering us on. If you work in sales, you know that you'll have to deal with a lot of rejection before you make enough sales to earn your commission. Many jobs require hours of tireless work before we see results, and often that work goes unrecognized. As adults, we rely on intrinsic motivation to succeed.

You have the power to teach your players how to dig deep and find inspiration inside themselves. Use drills and laps to help them do this. Talk to them about the satisfaction that comes from accomplishing a private, personal victory such as doing more push-ups than you asked or running faster than ever before or setting a personal rebound record.

Encourage your players to consider their previous accomplishments, set personal goals that they can measure and then push themselves to grow. Emphasize that private, personal victories are more important than victories seen out on the playing field. Once they experience the power of private victories, they will have a skill to reflect upon when they need internal motivation.

While you're working on intrinsic motivation, start training the players to act as mini-coaches. Tell them that you can't be everywhere at once and that you need them to encourage one another, build each other up, cheer each other on and inspire each other to be their very best. Remind them that you're not just a group of people trying to win a game. You are a team. A family! Then ask them to support and believe in each other.

Your enthusiasm will give them the power to find internal drive. When you tap into internal motivation, your players will become unstoppable.

Build Their Confidence
It's time for another story!

I had a young lady join my team when she was a sixth grader. She had potential, but needed a lot of attention to develop it into concrete skills. As I got to know her, I realized that her home life was not good. Because of the negativity she endured at home, she had no confidence in herself or her skills.

I concentrated on building her confidence, focusing on who she was on the inside. Not how many shots she could make, but how hard she tried, emphasizing how much I respected her character as she fought to improve. I praised effort, not results, and character, not accomplishments.

Once she began to realize what a wonderful young girl she was, it was easy to build her basic fundamental skills and take her to the next level. Today she is a confident (yet not cocky) young woman with skills that have high school coaches and AAU programs begging her to join their teams.

This is the challenge you have before you: to build the confidence of your players.

That confidence will help them succeed in all areas of life. Confident women choose better partners. They apply to higher-paying jobs. They are willing to take risks. Confidence makes the difference between landing a job or getting rejected. Teach your players this secret and you'll give them a magic key they will use for the rest of their lives.

Help Them Understand Terminology and Rules

Use practice and training time to teach your players to master everything about their craft, including the terminology. As they learn what moves and strategies are called, they will feel more capable out on the field. When properly educated, they can glean tips from other players, read up on the sport on their own and feel confident when they move up to another team.

This includes understanding rules, the calls the referee makes during the game and the specifics of fouls and violations. They need to understand the big picture of the game in order to play well. If you don't make sure they understand the rules, they will be hesitant on the court, afraid of getting called for a foul.

This also helps them internalize the idea that there are rules and terminology to be used in a specific arena. In the workplace, this is especially important to understand and respect. You set them up for success when you teach this principle.

Teach Them Court Sense (Teamwork)

You've met that person in the workplace who just doesn't get his or her role, right? The person who speaks out of turn in meetings, doesn't pull his or her weight or takes over entire projects, disregarding the input of co-workers?

That happens on sports teams, too, and it's your job to teach the players something I call court sense.

Court sense is the understanding of how the players on a team work together on the court to make efficient plays. You need to teach them the value of each position, including what is expected of each position on the court. Beyond this, they need to understand how each position contributes to the overall strength of the team and how particular plays work.

I advise you to teach every player how to play every position on the court. This empowers every through greater understanding of how her contributions mesh with the contributions of other team members, enabling each player to be more of an asset for the team.

Most importantly, this strategy helps every player understand the value of her teammates and responsibilities, obstacles to success, etc. The more the team understands the value of each player working together, the more the team will develop a true bond. This should be accomplished during practices since you will need each player to play their best position during the games. However, during practices you can help them understand the bigger picture.

Help Them to Learn Persistence Through Conditioning

I'm a basketball coach, so most of my examples are for basketball players. I'm not sure what sport you are teaching, but whatever it is, you need your players to be in good shape overall. This means you probably have them running, lifting weights or doing some other form of conditioning.

While all coaches have to crack the whip from time to time to get every player to work hard at conditioning, you will want to instill an appreciation for fitness and being in shape overall. Players learn persistence and endurance through conditioning challenges. Both of these character traits will carry them far in relationships, parenting and the workplace.

Show Them What Effective Communication Looks Like

While playing any team sport, you are taught to communicate on the court or field. Whether it's yelling, "I'm open!" or a nod of the head that lets your teammate know it's time to make a move, communication is essential.

Teach your players to communicate with each other on and off the court. Tell them exactly what you expect from them, giving specific examples. "Susan, when Kaelyn does X, you need to say Y and do Z." Then have them practice situations where they will need to communicate, critiquing their communication skills and then running the play again until they get it.

Something a lot of coaches don't talk about (but that I find important) is to teach your players how to communicate through body language (in addition to verbal communication skills). For example, when a coach or player is speaking, everyone on the team should maintain eye contact and upright posture showing that they are fully engaged in the conversation. Do not allow players to slouch, look away or otherwise disrespect whomever is speaking.

Communication is one of the most important and lasting skills you can teach a player. It can save a marriage; it is essential for problem solving. Communication skills are necessary for interviewing, performing well on the job, negotiating changes and managing others. These skills are required for any relationship, including the parent-child relationship.

Teach your players to communicate and you've taught them how to survive in this world.

The Power of Effective Training

You may have thought of training as "just practices," but I hope you now see the incredible potential of those practice sessions.

As one of my players' parents commented, "Coach teaches life first and basketball second. She teaches the ladies about confidence, hard work and winning on and off the court." (Thank you, Timothy, for the positive review!)

You can make a difference by investing yourself fully in the training of the young women on your team. Coach in a conscious manner, making an impact on the girls that will last a lifetime.

Chapter Four: Good Offense — On the Court and In Life

As I teach my players good offensive strategies and skills, I like to imagine I am preparing them to take full advantage of every opportunity that will come their way in life. Just like they shoot for a basket, they can shoot for dreams and to accomplish goals. They are learning how to be assertive and get what they want in life.

This part of the game is usually the most intuitive part for the players; after all, everybody knows that you have to move forward if you want to win a game. And yet, you'll be surprised at how many girls are hesitant once on the court. They know (in their head) what they are supposed to do, but often lack the assertiveness to make the play happen.

It's your job to teach them offensive strategies and to empower them with the confidence to act on those strategies. Once you combine these two factors, your girls will be unstoppable.

The following are things I teach my basketball players that translate into life skills long after they stop playing on my team. You may need to open your mind to determine which analogous skills you teach your sports team, but basically, these are offensive moves and skills that will help a young woman assert herself in life.

Train Them to Work as a Team — Passing and Catching

Although you probably do not think about it, you pass the ball a lot in your everyday life. When you delegate work while working on a team project or managing a team, you pass the ball. You also need to be able to catch when your manager and/or co-workers delegate work to you. Even when working on a goal with your spouse, you both pass and catch the ball as needed. Really, life is a game of passing and catching as we work our way through challenges together.

No team wins a basketball game without players knowing how to pass well. This is a skill you will want to practice up and down the court until it is second nature to your players. Then, during scrimmages, you need to help your players realize the power of passing instead of trying to one-woman it down the court.

I once had a young girl who joined my team when she was in fifth grade. This young lady was the star player in her grade and used to do it all on the court, but she did not like to pass. She had skills, but she was not a team player.

A lot of coaches would have just let her have her way, but I knew that her resistance to passing and working with her teammates would hurt the team as a whole. I parked her on the bench and explained to her that she had to show me she was willing to pass and work with her teammates if she wanted to see any playing time. After a few months of sitting on the bench and a lot of frustration, she decided to try to work within my program. She is now a great team player who has led her team to championships both locally and nationally.

Show Them the Value of Control — Ball Handling & Dribbling

In life and in basketball, you have to learn how to control the ball and move it forward. You can't wait for the basket to magically come to you; you have to move the ball down the court without losing control to the opposition.

In life, you need to do the same thing. Very few goals can be accomplished in one swift move. To get out of debt, you have to establish a plan and stick with it without getting distracted. To finish a project, you have to break it down into small pieces and finish each piece in turn without losing sight of the end goal. To lose weight, you have to tackle diet and exercise and stick with them to see progress.

In basketball, we run drills called base running which teach players to move towards the opportunity, attack the basket and not wait for the opportunity to come to them. This drill helps them build courage and self-confidence that they can control the ball, moving it down the court to the eventual goal.

Teach Them to Shoot and Score

Naturally, every player wants to learn how to make a basket; it's the main goal of the game. It is the most recognized piece of the offense in the game of basketball; it's where all the glory is.

In basketball, we practice the following:

- Lay-ups
- Free-throws
- Jump shots
- Hook shots

While you may have to adapt this section to apply to your particular sport, I have provided examples of what I teach my players in regards to these specific basketball moves. While we work on these basketball skills, I weave in stories of how these skills translate into life skills. You will want to do the same with your players.

Lay-ups

Lay-ups are made by leaping from below, laying the ball up near the basket and using one hand to bounce it off the backboard and into the basket. It is the closest shot and the easiest way to score in a game.

The life lesson associated with this move is this: you get many easy opportunities in life that can place you closer to your goals. You just need to take advantage of them and score.

Free-throws

Forget everything you know about your shot when it comes to free throws; it's a different state of mind. It's the only uncontested and stationary shot in the game. When you get to shoot free-throws, you need to operate like a well-positioned, well-lubricated machine with every shot.

Free-throws are not "free" "throws," they are "earned" "shots" that earn you points. This is the type of shot that takes the most work because it's a *mental* shot.

Many times in life you will come across opportunities where there is no one in your way except yourself. You get into your own mind and convince yourself that you are unable to do something. Teach your players to win the mental game. Teach them to override self-doubt and to encourage themselves that they can do it.

Jump shots

Players who learn how to shoot and score get the satisfaction of knowing they can make a difference on a team.

The confidence they gain from this experience sets them up to believe that they can also score in life — whether that be asking someone out on a date, applying for a challenging job, tackling a difficult project or making a difference in their community. When you teach a girl to shoot and score, you teach her that she can succeed.

Hook shots

This is when you attempt to make a basket by jumping, typically while an opponent is in front of you. The offensive player, usually turned perpendicular to the basket, gently throws the ball with a sweeping motion of her arm in an upward arc with a follow-through that ends over her head.

Sometimes obstacles/people will get in your way of your goal. You might have to jump over them to achieve your goals. There are times in life when you will need to go in a different direction to meet your goal.

Make Sure They Know How to Move — Cutting and Faking

Life doesn't always progress in a straight line, on schedule. As you well know, we all hit obstacles when we set out to achieve goals. It is essential that we learn how to adapt to situations.

In basketball, we use sliding, cutting and faking to move around the court and do what you have to do to free yourself up for an opportunity. When a girl learns how to get open for a pass on the court, she's learning how to assertively get herself out of a jam in real life.

Encourage Them to Support Others — Pick/Screen and Roll

Sometimes we get to be the star player; sometimes we don't. In many situations, we have to support the project lead or our spouse in ways that might feel less rewarding.

As your players practice pick/screen and roll drills, they are learning to assist other players in an essential way. As they help their teammates get the ball down the court, they also watch for their opportunity to jump in and rebound or score, if needed.

These skills translate into the workforce since we all have times when we need to complete our part of the project as we support and then jump in when needed at a more intense capacity. When a young woman learns this, she is prepared for the real dynamics of life.

Teach Them to Never Say Never — Rebounding, Jumping and Boxing Out

Have you ever attempted to achieve a goal only to be blocked by negativity or unfortunate circumstances? People who succeed know how to handle discouragement and obstacles so that they can try again and again, persevering until they succeed.

I teach my basketball players the value of the rebound, jumping and boxing out. You may fail at your first shot, but if you get the rebound, you get another chance to score. If your teammate misses and you get the rebound, your team has another chance to score. If you jump and tip the ball out of a competitor's hand, you also give your team another chance to score. If you position yourself in the best spot to get the rebound by "boxing out" — i.e., by positioning yourself between an opponent and the basket and maintaining body contact with the player you guarding — you also can increase your chances of scoring.

All of these moves increase your team's chances of scoring.

A Good Offense Moves the Ball Forward

As a coach, you have the opportunity to teach these young women how to move the ball forward on the court and how to believe in their abilities to move forward in life.

As one parent commented, "Coach LaShun's service and professionalism goes above and beyond one's expectations. She sacrifices her time to see others succeed. She has dedicated herself to help others become well-rounded individuals, incorporating their personal, professional and spiritual growth in the process." (Thank you, Scooter, for the positive review!)

You, too, can be the coach who makes a lasting difference!

Chapter Five: A Good Defense is as Important as a Good Offense

I personally love the saying that "a good defense wins games and championships" because I've seen it happen again and again. I also love the quote (from one of my favorite movies, *Love and Basketball*): "Offense sells tickets; defense wins games."

Sure, scoring is fun. Everyone wants to score. That's because most of the cheering comes when points are scored. However, anyone who knows basketball knows that a solid defense is what prevents the other team from burying you.

It takes a certain mentality to think of defense first, but that mentality can set a young woman up for success in life. Defensive training can be used to overcome obstacles because it gives you the mindset of always persevering and never giving up. We do not have control over everything that happens to us, but we can change the way we defend against the problems and obstacles that come our way.

Another way of thinking about defense is to realize how important it is to be able to adapt to challenges. In a game, you have to adapt and change to handle whatever comes at you. Are you dealing with aggressive opponents who break the rules (and a referee who isn't calling fouls)? Is one of your teammates off her game that day and in need of extra support? Does the other team have a fast and skilled offensive player?

As you play defense, you need to be ready to adjust to whatever comes at you — often with little or no advance notice.

In life, you also need to defend the things that are important to you. Just like you have to defend the basketball hoop, you also have to defend your job, reputation, character, family and rights as a human being.

Good defense doesn't just win games. It helps you win in life.

Teach Them How to Remain Standing — Footwork

As adults, we face challenges, some of which are incredibly daunting. A project manager doesn't believe in you. A request for a loan is denied. A family member bad-mouths you to your spouse.

When faced with tricky situations, we have to find ways around the obstacles. We get up each morning. We decide to go after the things that are important to us like a promotion, a new job, a date, etc. Instead of sitting on the sidelines and letting life pass us by, we actively pursue the things we desire.

On the court, players have to learn how to keep moving so they can get around obstacles and avoid getting blocked. As players learn how to do the footwork necessary to get free, they learn what it takes to work their way around obstacles in life.

In basketball we practice pivoting and the jab step. Adapt this concept to your sport and emphasize the advantage of continuous movement. If the player is moving, the opposition can't lock her down. Yes, it is exhausting to continuously move, but the advantages of being mobile far outweigh the problems that occur when a player just stands rooted to the ground.

Help Them Understand How Boxing Out Gives Them the Upper Hand

When someone attempts to approach you with negativity to create problems in your life, you have to block the negativity, right?

In basketball, players learn how to box out opponents to prevent them from getting the ball or the advantage. Practice boxing out by putting your players against each other in scrimmages, showcasing how effective this move is. Then talk to them about how this form of offensive defense also works in real life.

In most situations, if we pay attention, we can anticipate potential problems. If we "box out" in our real life situations, we can prevent problems from becoming too big simply by taking control of the situation. You might schedule a meeting with your boss before a bigger meeting to make sure you see eye-to-eye (rather than risk getting humiliated in front of the whole group because you assumed things would go well). You might recognize that your project has a potential obstacle and remove it before you try to progress. Boxing out is an anticipatory move that gives you the upper hand.

Show Them to Recover Lost Opportunities by Getting the Rebound

Too often, people think failure is final.

They fail the bar exam and they never try again. They get divorced and refuse to date again. They give up because failure crushes them.

Train your girls to see failure as an opportunity to try again. Inspire them to learn how to get the rebounds in life, even when their first attempts don't get the results desired.

A Good Defense Never Gives Up

You've been there. You are in a meeting and no one seems to be listening to you. Your nemesis not only tries to derail your project, but he cuts you off when you try to take the platform. That is when you box him out and prepare yourself for a rebound, which is your opportunity to grab the ball and shoot, putting the ball in the basket to score.

Teach your girls good defense and they'll use it for the rest of their lives.

Chapter Six: The Games — Seeing the Results of Your Hard Work

After weeks of pre-season training and conditioning, it is "game time!" Your players have to put all of the training, offense and defense skills to the test. Your players get to showcase their talent, just as you would after you interviewed for a position, landed the job and started your first day at work. You now are on the court in front of your boss and co-workers to let them see your talent and character.

Everyone who wants to achieve real success has to work hard, which is something you learn when playing any competitive sport. The following chapter details how game time trains young women to succeed in real life when it's time to perform.

Teach Them to Perform Under Pressure

It's one thing to dribble down the court and shoot a basket when you're scrimmaging against your teammates; it's a lot harder when you're playing against skilled opponents with a drive to win. This is when your players learn how to put aside their anxieties and perform.

Game time is one of the best preparations for real life. When these young women get their first real jobs and have to give presentations or that first sales call, they will remember how it felt to catch the ball and make a basket. When they bring home their infant who starts crying, they will remember how they endured long runs even though they felt like giving up. Thanks to their time in games, they will know that they can dig deep and find inner strength to perform when necessary. That knowledge will help them become amazingly inspirational adults who find success.

Show Them How to Keep Their Cool

Some of your opponents won't play by the rules. Maybe the ref doesn't make all the calls she should; maybe the players on the other team are big and rough. Parents might yell from the sidelines. The other coach might say derogatory things about your team.

You get to show these young women how to hold their heads high and play with dignity, regardless of how fair or unfair the playing field is.

Your example will teach them how to handle injustice in the real world. In the workforce, they will experience discrimination and co-workers who want to take credit for their work. At home, they will deal with crabby partners who had bad days. You are teaching them how to remain composed and calm in the face of adversity, a skill that will help them handle difficult situations with grace and strength.

Instill the Value of Time Management

You've learned the value of managing your time both through your own experiences and by watching other people who struggle with it, right? We've all been burned by a coworker who doesn't complete projects on time or partners who make us miss plane flights or don't pay the bills on time, costing us late fees and embarrassment.

As a coach, you get to teach players how to be independent and how to manage their time in a way that is respectful of others and shows both support and respect for the team as a whole.

You can do this by emphasizing the importance of:
- Getting to practice on time.
- Putting jackets/clothes/shoes in bags and lining them up nicely.
- Turning off phones during practice.
- Contacting you (coach) regarding missing practices/games.

It's tempting to let players blame parents and even other players instead of taking personal responsibility, but you only hurt them when you do this. Instead of communicating just with the parents, you will want to:
- Give players your email and cell phone number.
- Send out all communications to both players and their parents and make it clear that the players are the ones responsible, not the parents.
- Hold the players accountable for lateness, missed practices/games and lack of communication.
- Talk about how lateness/absences affect the whole team so they understand the ways their actions affect other people.
- Talk about ways to overcome problems with transportation, irresponsible parents (without saying anything offensive), etc. Show them how to find solutions when the people around them are not reliable.

As you teach your players to be proactive, independent and responsible, you equip them with life skills that will help them get and keep jobs and become responsible members of society. These skills are essential, and many kids don't learn them at home.

Help Them Understand What Really Matters

Remember those personal private victories?

Those are what you need to emphasize, especially when your team loses.

Win or lose, did you play your best?

Win or lose, did you have a personal victory?

Even if you failed today, will you pick yourself up again tomorrow and try harder?

If the answers are yes, then you have succeeded as a coach.

Now that you're thinking this way, it's easy to see how the skills on the court translate into skills in real life, isn't it? This is why coaching is so much more than keeping kids off the streets or spending extra time with your kids. Coaching is an opportunity to make a real difference in the lives of young women. It's a chance to make your mark in this world.

Conclusion: Are You In or Out?

I know coaching isn't easy.

I've been tempted to quit. At one point, the personal losses felt like they were too much. Political pressure from other coaches or parents got me down. I thought about giving up.

But I stuck with it.

Why?

At that time in my life, as I was considering quitting, a Bears player became an assistant coach for a kid for whom I had become a legal guardian. This wonderful girl introduced me to the Bears player as her mom, and in that awkward moment, I had to clarify that I was the "Coach Mom," not the biological mom. I also mentioned something about how I had coached her team, but didn't think I would coach much longer.

The Bears player looked me in the eye and said, "You can't quit. I know more about you as 'Coach Mom' than I know about most of these kids' biological parents. You are making a difference."

That did it. I stuck with coaching because I realized these kids needed me.

These girls need YOU.

You don't know it yet, but you're about to change lives.

The skills you teach these girls can be applied to daily life. Whether you win or lose the individual games, you can teach these young women how to win in life. That is most important of all.

Warmly,
Coach R LaShun Williams

Would you *please* do me a favor?

If you found **Throw Like A Girl: How Good Coaches Transform Girls Into Successful Women** useful please consider posting a short review on Amazon and/or Goodreads. Word of mouth is an author's best friend and much appreciated. It will only take a minute, and would really help me get the word out about my book.

Would you like personal coaching? Want to tell me what the next version of this book should include? Visit **www.YourLifeDestiny.com.**

Sources

11 Facts About Teens and Self Esteem. (n.d.). Retrieved June 18, 2016, from https://www.dosomething.org/us/facts/11-facts-about-teens-and-self-esteem

Statistics on Girls & Women's Self Esteem, Pressures & Leadership Heart of Leadership. (n.d.). Retrieved June 18, 2016, from http://www.heartofleadership.org/statistics/

Daley, S. (1991, January 9). Little Girls Lose Their Self-Esteem Way to Adolescence, Study Finds. *The New York Times.*

Psychological and Social Benefits of Playing True Sport. (n.d.). Retrieved June 18, 2016, from http://truesport.org/resources/publications/reports/psychological-and-social-benefits-of-playing-true-sport/

Casey, M. (2014). Want to succeed in business? Then play high school sports. Retrieved June 18, 2016, from http://fortune.com/2014/06/19/high-school-sports-business-cornell-job-market/

Segelken, H. R. (2014, June 14). Youth sports 'spill over' to career success | Cornell Chronicle. Retrieved June 18, 2016, from http://news.cornell.edu/stories/2014/06/youth-sports-spill-over-career-success

Ford, L. (2014, February 13). New Report: Majority of U.S. Teens Don't Live in Intact Families. Retrieved June 18, 2016, from http://dailysignal.com/2014/02/13/new-report-majority-u-s-teens-dont-live-intact-families/

Dove's "Campaign for Real Beauty" helps to promote self-esteem in young women (video). (2010, August 27). Retrieved June 18, 2016, from
http://www.examiner.com/article/dove-s-campaign-for-real-beauty-helps-to-promote-self-esteem-young-women-video

About the Author

Rebecca L. Williams "Coach RLaShun" is a well-known and highly respected as a basketball coach has spent over two decades coaching and training youth basketball. She graduated in 1996 from Gustavus Adolphus College with a BA in Pre-Law / Psychology. She has over 20 years of experience as a Professional Consulting within the Human Resource field. Having a strong passion for coaching others towards success, she also obtained a Professional Coaching Certification and have been an Ambassador for the International Coaching Academy (ICA) and owned her own Coaching Practice, Your Life Destiny for over 20 years coaching individuals towards their success. She coaches companies and adults towards their success, yet she also spends a lot of her time coaching our youth. For more information regarding her life coaching services visit: **www.YourLifeDestiny.com.**

www.ingramcontent.com/pod-product-compliance
Lightning Source LLC
Chambersburg PA
CBHW060635280326
41933CB00012B/2051